The Gifts of Gratitude

A New Paradigm Using the Gift of Gratitude

Theresa M. Ross, Ph.D.

DEDICATION

This book is dedicated to all the teachers of wisdom who surrounded me with love and spiritual knowledge. I am especially grateful to Oriental and Zinnie for introducing me to the Divine and many great master teachers. Both taught me to always look for good in all life experiences.

TABLE OF CONTENTS

INTRODUCTION

Life has many positive rewards that can be viewed as gifts when we express gratitude. It helps us in many ways and multiplies when it is repeatedly demonstrated. When we have made a concerted effort to be grateful, we focus on the good things in our lives. Yet, there are also times that cause us to experience something that we deem not good. However, with a shift in perception, we can gleam parts of what's considered not so good as having a golden nugget, revealing something positive that was not noticed before.

For example, you lose your job and become upset, but in reviewing your skills, you discover you can start your own business or move into a different area of employment. Many things can help us in our practice of thankfulness. We will begin by defining gratitude and its significance in our lives. Then, we will look at the gifts it gives us and discover how our mindset, health, well-being, self-gratitude, journaling, colors, mindfulness, exercise, and several other disciplines help develop the practice of gratitude. The gifts that gratitude brings to the disciplines stated are immense and helpful in finding the inner sanctuary where the authentic you resides.

We start, however, with the significance of your mindset. The observance of how you view your life experiences helps you to begin perceiving how you are receiving and labeling what comes to you. How often do you observe positive feedback? Or do you observe only experiences primarily as negative? You will examine your mindset to understand its place in the thankful arena. During this time of profound social, economic, political, and technological shifts, we are faced with many adverse reports about our world. Placing a mirror on the events of the world today, we observe that the mirror reflects stress and disharmony, and shows a lack of love for self and others and a lack of listening and communication that allows for understanding.

Love and gratitude for yourself and others have taken a back seat to many of the daily negatives. Some individuals, in many instances, have fallen victim to a herd mentality, a mentality where they follow the crowd to fit into society and gain a sense of belonging.

There is a real need for individuals to begin to take inventory of their behavior and their feelings about themselves. Self-examination means understanding what you say to yourself and others, how you feel about yourself, and the behaviors you express. Inquiry becomes an absolute necessity if there is to be a change in individual consciousness that extends to society to make it a safe environment. Everyone should try to bring thankfulness into their life to receive the gifts that it has to offer.

In the words of Camille Sacco, we find words that speak to the need for self-examination. Sacco says: "Your outer world is a direct reflection of your inner world. If you want to change the world you see, start working on your inner world."

As an educator, life coach, and ordained minister, I have encouraged and inspired those who feel discouraged and think that they are not valued or have a sense of not belonging. I have given them words of encouragement to help them place value on themselves. One of the gifts of gratitude is learning to love yourself just the way you are. I have shared wisdom that enabled them to seek internal guidance and to claim their power of self by realizing their uniqueness.

I speak from a place of authority about the benefits of gratitude. I have learned that if you want or need to change your life or the life of someone else, you will find that words of love, kindness, appreciation, and upliftment will work wonders in helping you to do so.

This book on the Gifts of Gratitude will give guidance on the ways that you can begin the process of learning who you are and how the emotion of gratitude can change the way you feel, improve relationships, have a positive impact on your health, help to gain trust and honesty in yourself and reduce stress by understanding that your actions are yours to own. You will learn that you hold power and are no longer at the mercy of others. The journey starts with honesty and a gratitude mindset.

One of the hardest things in life is to take a hard look in the mirror and observe and appreciate who you are as a person. The journey begins with learning about and understanding the disciplines that help you to experience gratefulness. These disciplines can be found within the pages of this book. The surprise waiting for you can be found in gratitude, healthy living, well-being, self-gratitude, colors, journaling and so much more.

"When you arise in the morning, think of what a precious privilege it is to be alive, to breathe, to think, to enjoy, to love." Marcus Aurelius

Chapter 1

GRATITUDE

It has only been recently that gratitude became the subject of scientific research. Dr. Emmons, an expert on gratitude and its benefits, states that appreciation can contribute significantly to an individual's life, making a big difference.

Gratitude offers many gifts, and science has supported it. When practiced regularly, it provides benefits that can be measured. The benefits include physical, psychological, and interpersonal ones.

For example, when people change their attitude about themselves and their lives, they shift in how they interact with others, which becomes more pleasurable. The shift causes better feelings about oneself, and this is extended to other people. We could say that pleasant feelings become contagious.

The definition of gratitude, as defined by Webster's New Collegiate Dictionary, is "the state of being grateful" or of thankfulness. It is one of many positive emotions.

The derivatives of this Latin root connect to the words, kindness, generousness, gifts, and the beauty of giving and receiving or getting something for nothing. This definition covers the way in which gratitude is expressed.

The practice of gratitude can bring on a good feeling and be a stimulus for motivation to complete tasks or goals that need to be finished. When the goodness in life is acknowledged, gratitude is at the forefront of that goodness, and life takes on the purpose of living. It is more than a politeness or a superficial feeling.

The best way to practice gratitude is to have a daily routine that includes reminding yourself of the gifts that come to you, the grace and benefits received, and the things you enjoy. Gratefulness allows you to give affirmation to the goodness in your life. One of the ways to practice is to use a gratitude journal to capture the gifts that gratitude brings you. It allows you to perceive the meaning of events in your life. Writing about your experiences gives you an opportunity to reflect on them and bring, once again, the feelings that surfaced within you. Many feelings that surfaced are like a beautiful flower from a seed. The experiences that you find and explore can give you challenging new meanings as you transform your perception into that of gratefulness. A perception that recognizes the good in your life without minimizing or denying the challenges or hardships that are also present.

At first, you may notice that writing about your gratefulness may be discouraging because you are searching for and trying to remember all that is good in your life. However, as you continue the practice, you will find that the more you count your blessings, the more blessings you will have to write in your journal. In writing to capture your benefits and gifts, you will no longer take them for granted in your life.

The elements in your life that you are grateful for can be considered gifts. The gift of gratitude contributes to greater feelings of positiveness, better mood, and acceptance of experiences you encounter. Its gift is given without reservation, whether you notice it or not. When noticed you are rewarded positively.

Make a habit of practicing gratitude and observe the things you are grateful for daily. The more you practice, the more it becomes easier to see the good in your experiences. What may have seemed like too little will be viewed as more than enough.

The Roman philosopher, Cicero said, "Gratitude is not only the greatest of virtues, but the parent of all others."

Chapter 2

A GRATITUDE MINDSET

Catching Thoughts Before They Misbehave

Let's begin the journey of exploring the gifts of gratitude and see how these gifts can change your life. A gift is defined as the act, right, or power of giving. Gratitude helps you with a positive attitude, gives a sense of peace, improves relationships, impacts your health and well-being, and lets you move beyond isolation. You gain in many ways when you practice the art of gratitude.

As a grateful person, you will be shifted from negative self-talk to positive talk of being thankful. Your internal dialogue will not be the same. The language of gratitude makes it easy for you to be thankful for the support you receive from family, friends, and people you encounter during your daily experiences. It becomes easier to recognize the good streaming into your life when you acknowledge the kindness extended to you. Awareness of kindness will bring about good feelings that you will want to experience more than once.

You might ask, "Does gratitude matter?" And the answer is a resounding yes. Gratitude does matter. There is evidence showing that gratitude matters. According to Dr. Emmons, gratitude enhances nearly every area of your life, and it is in ample supply because it is accessible and available to everyone.

No age barriers or status requirements exist for a life lived in gratitude. Whatever your thoughts are about gratitude, this book will give you a new perspective and the tools to improve your life using the gifts of appreciation. You will move from a space of dissatisfaction with your life to one of excitement, being energized, with a feeling of power.

By re-educating your mind, you will discover that your awareness of small experiences dramatically affects how you feel and view life. Gratitude is different from the positive emotions of hope and optimism. Although each one of them has a position with the positive aspects of life.

Hope and optimism are expectations for the future and the ability to recognize avenues through which positive outcomes may be achieved. There are no expectations attached to gratitude. An appreciation of the positive aspects of life in the present moment fundamentally characterizes gratitude. This kind of appreciation does not necessarily involve being thankful for the support given by others. Several everyday experiences may be described as giving you a chance to express gratitude. Those experiences may include an appreciation of the beauty of a sunset or thankfulness for the experience of taking a walk in the park and observing the beauty of the environment.

When you have a positive attitude and feelings about life, gratitude affects your well-being.

Several research studies found that gratitude had a medium to a largely positive relationship with multiple elements of psychological well-being, including environmental mastery, personal growth, positive relationships, the purpose of life, and self-acceptance. In addition, in these studies, it was found that several of the areas studied were not dependent on social interactions. Gratitude contributed to the attainment of happiness or eudaemonic as compared to hedonics or pleasure. Thus, the satisfaction of life is tied to experiences that you appreciate.

My experience of being aware of gratitude's place in life came about when I moved away from family and friends to attend college. I moved to another state that had no relatives in the area that I could visit and establish family bonds; however, I was fortunate to meet a wonderful friend and mentor, Zinnie, who took me under her wings, giving me love, support and making me a part of her family.

Zinnie would tell me, "Never refuse an experience; always be in an acceptance mode. Look for the golden treasure in the middle of all that comes to you. The good and the not-so-good. Gratitude will help you discover the treasure hidden inside of you." The many lessons she taught me led to the development of a new mindset about life experiences.

She also introduced me to many great philosophers whose teachings focused on the power of thoughts and the way they create in one's life. The introduction to these philosophers helped me to understand that my thoughts and beliefs had a lot to do with how I felt and to notice people and things that I attracted in my life. The teachings of these philosophers enabled me to have successful outcomes in my education, relationships, and family. I learned that a change in attitude about the experiences I encountered would be less stressful if I developed an attitude of gratitude.

Awareness of how you think is essential in understanding gratitude's power. As you go through your day, many thoughts might surface as you think about events and experiences. But how are you interpreting them?

For example, some thoughts focus on memories, while others focus on current issues and situations. Still, other ideas might be attached to future happenings. Learn to be aware of your thoughts; you can replace those that do not serve you well, those that cause emotional disturbances, and judgmental thoughts, with those that bring joy and tranquility.

When looking at negative thoughts, you will find that they cause misconceptions about situations and make you jump to conclusions that are not based on the reality of a problem. Ruminations are often chronic and outside of your awareness. The power of gratitude helps in changing your mental perspective.

However, your thoughts can also inspire you and help you to see and feel grateful for all that is good in your life. They can, in many instances, change your perception of what you think of as terrible. Although there will be challenges and difficulties, choosing thankful thoughts can sometimes make a difference in how you process them.

When you become an observer of your thoughts, you can begin to eliminate and block incoming negative thoughts.

As an observer, you will see your thoughts without judging them. If you do not give energetic strength to them, they will quiet down and eventually disappear.

To be grateful, you must realize that gratefulness has more to do with managing your thoughts and looking for the good in situations, experiences, and people. A feeling of joy will be experienced when you are liberated from ungrateful and judgmental thoughts. There is an old African proverb that says, "If you can overcome the enemy on the inside, the enemy on the outside won't be able to do you any harm." The enemy within can be daily ungrateful thoughts rehearsed or replayed constantly within your mind. You are looking for an experience of gratitude when you change your mind, along with gratitude's benefits.

To change your thinking, you must change what goes into your mind. According to Dr. Bruce Lipton, you must examine the consequences of energy invested in your thinking. Thinking is the mind's energy source for helping you change your life.

It's essential to monitor where the brain's energy is expended since there is a relationship between your conscious and unconscious mind. The conscious mind is creative and can produce positive and inspirational thoughts. The subconscious mind, however, is a bank of stimulus-response tapes derived from instincts and learned experiences. Since it is habitual, it will continually play the same behavioral responses to life's signals. Therefore, observing and monitoring the surface behavioral responses is crucial.

Self-image plays a role in the development of a grateful attitude. The world around you can be interpreted based on how you describe yourself. Your picture of yourself and your environment affects your perceptions and interpretations of the world around you. A poor self-image distorts messages received from people, and the way life events are perceived and interpreted. If you feel ungrateful, the ungratefulness can feed off itself to create more ungratefulness.

Therefore, become aware of your self-talk, the constant stream of unspoken thoughts. It can weaken or strengthen how you feel about yourself. Most self-talk is destructive because of the focus on what is wrong rather than ideas for improving things. Too much negative self-talk for an extended period can lead to ungratefulness, anxiety, and potentially depression.

When there is positive self-talk, your mood will improve, causing you to have a greater appreciation for all that appears in your life.

Recognizing the power of your thoughts is a move toward mastery of internal dialogue, your interaction with people, and your environment. You have the power and ability to be grateful for your physical, emotional, and intellectual experiences. Learn to love yourself and appreciate your uniqueness. Love yourself enough to have a state of mind that allows you to accept the gifts of gratitude and be satisfied with your life.

Change your words, and you can change your world. Improve your comments, and you can improve your world.

Changing your mindset, however, can take time and requires patience. The reason for this is due to your mind being beautifully designed to react automatically. Your brain and nervous system build "highways" for paths of information that make things like thought patterns somewhat automatic. The challenge with this elegant system of ease is that if you want to change the direction of the flow of your neurological pattern, there must be consistency because it takes practice and rethinking against your hard wiring.

It can be difficult to gain momentum after something goes wrong. But having the ability to rebound, strengthen your heart, and have the determination to survive gives you an opportunity to recognize your resilience.

You will find that you have everything within you to meet the challenges that life brings to you. You will be inspired to meet your days with hope and courage. And with a new mindset, your future will be brighter.

"Embrace gratitude and do not be surprised when your life makes a shift in a new direction."

Theresa M. Ross

"Expressing gratitude can be as simple as seeing a hummingbird take nectar from a flower, causing you to vocalize 'Oh how beautiful, what a majestic scene.'"

Theresa M. Ross

Chapter 3

HEALTHY LIVING

Feeling Good from Lifestyle Changes

When it comes to health and wellness, everyone agrees that being sick is not something they look forward to. Especially if the illness causes them to be nonfunctional, and unable to do daily activities. There is no rush to join the medical and pharmaceutical community. It is in the interest of all to do whatever is necessary to be an outlier when it comes to health and wellness.

Health is defined as a state of complete emotional and physical well-being. When you can handle stress, you can live a longer, more active life and will find that good health becomes a central theme in your life.

The World Health Organization, in 1948, defined health in terms still used by modern authorities today:

"Health is a state of complete physical, mental, social well-being and not merely the absence of disease or infirmity."

The World Health Organization (WHO) clarified the definition of health even more in 1986. They stated that health is:

"A resource for everyday life, not the objective of living. Health is a positive concept emphasizing social and personal resources as well as physical capacities." Rather than an end, health becomes a resource to support your societal function. Your life becomes meaningful and purposeful when you have a healthy lifestyle.

When you have good physical health, your body functions will operate at their peak. Good physical health includes regular exercise, balanced nutrition, and adequate rest. A healthy lifestyle also promotes physical well-being. When you maintain physical fitness, you will gain the protection of your heart functions, and muscular strength, giving you flexibility, and better composition of your body.

There is a relationship between good physical health and mental health, which can improve the quality of your life. According to the US Department of Health and Human Services, mental health refers to emotional, social, and psychological well-being. It is as important as your physical health which is part of an active lifestyle. The absence of depression, anxiety, or other disorders is not the only criterion for defining good mental health. Good mental health also depends on your ability to enjoy life, bounce back after difficult experiences, adapt to adversity, feel safe and secure, and achieve your full potential.

The ability to give thanks for good and not-so-good experiences dramatically affects the quality of your health, well-being, and life. When you can focus on what you are grateful for, you will find that gratitude offers gifts with great merit. When you are thankful, you may reflect on all that has been good in your life. Most research tends to focus on the positives of gratitude. However, gratitude isn't always about positive things in life. You are encouraged to be thankful for all the experiences that life has to offer. There is often an invisible blessing hiding in an experience that you do not like.

Research suggests that gratitude may be associated with numerous benefits, including better physical and psychological health. Two of the benefits are an increase in life satisfaction and happiness. In addition, several research studies suggest that you experience better health if you are grateful. In contrast, other research indicates that scientifically designed practices to increase gratitude can benefit your health and encourage you to adopt healthier habits.

A research study, conducted in 1995, found that participants who felt appreciation, an emotion related to gratitude, had their heart rate variability improved. Glenn Fox, Ph.D., a neuroscientist, states, "The limits of gratitude's health benefits are really in how much you pay attention to feeling and practicing gratitude. The more you practice gratitude, the easier it becomes for you to practice it when needed." Also, when you are grateful, you will sleep better.

Sleep and Gratitude

Researchers at the University of Manchester studied how gratitude influences sleep. The participants were given questionnaires to determine their level of gratitude and to measure their sleep performance. The researchers found that appreciation resulted in more positive and fewer negative thoughts before bedtime. In addition, the results showed a positive impact on sleep quality and duration.

We have all experienced a time when we cannot sleep because the mind is on speed dial and repeats something that did not go well over the day.

A worry might even become stuck in your mind. If a practice of gratitude is developed before bedtime, it can switch the thoughts in your mind to positive reviews and help you drift off into a deep restful sleep. Wayne Dyer, an American self-help author, stated, "If you focus on what you are grateful for before you go to sleep, then that is what you will marinate overnight." The expression of gratitude has a definite impact on your sleep.

Since sleep deprivation affects the body, gratitude practice before sleep can be beneficial. Getting ready for a restful night's sleep begins with reducing the day's activities. Use the time before going to bed to read or do something quiet and relaxing, setting the tone for an attitude of gratitude. Conversations with family members and friends should center around topics other than those focusing on controversial subjects.

Your sleep environment should be free of electronic equipment, i.e., computers, television, cell phones, and other items that emit blue light. When you retire for the evening, make sure that you turn off all lights and have windows covered to make the room dark. Good ventilation will help you have a restful night's sleep. Try to fall asleep within 10 minutes after retiring and sleep through the night.

Remember that sleep is a therapeutic activity that prepares you for the next day's activities. When you lack sleep, you will be impaired and not function at your best.

The practice of gratitude before falling asleep enhances the quality of sleep that you will have during the night.

Practicing gratitude is known to improve psychological health or well-being. It reduces many toxic emotions you might experience, such as envy, resentment, frustration, and regret. Robert Emmons, a leading gratitude researcher, has conducted many studies on the link between gratitude and well-being. His research affirms that appreciation effectively decreases depression and increases happiness. Some studies found that people who consciously count their blessings are happier and less depressed.

Those who are grateful get more sleep each night and spend less time awake before falling asleep. And grateful people feel more refreshed when they awaken.

As you begin each new day, remain quiet and feel a sense of gratitude for the evening rest, even if you did not get an adequate amount of sleep. Let gratitude be the theme for the day.

Food and Gratitude

There are several additional ways to cultivate more gratitude in your life. One of the ways includes practicing gratitude at mealtimes. Beginning with silently thanking a Higher Power and the people responsible for the food on your dinner plate. These include farmers, harvesters, and transporters of food to grocery stores for purchase.

Taking a moment to express gratitude for the food on your plate is a simple practice that reconnects you with the origins of your food. It also allows you to think about and be grateful to the individuals who harvested the food.

Food has a significant influence on your feelings of gratitude. Balanced meals help to maintain a positive outlook on life, which in turn can help you be more grateful for the blessings that come your way.

Eating foods high in nutrients, such as fruits and vegetables, can help you feel more energized and alert. In addition, healthy foods can help you be more productive, leading to a greater appreciation of your current possessions and things to come. One of the diets that you might explore is a plant-based diet. Along with eating fruits and vegetables, you would include nuts, seeds, whole grains, legumes, and beans. Plant-based foods improve the alkalinity of the body and help with gut health.

On the other hand, eating foods high in sugar and unhealthy fats can increase inflammation in the body. These foods can also cause you to be lazy and unmotivated. Unhealthy food can make it harder to feel grateful for the food you are consuming because of the way it makes you feel. High-fructose foods can make it difficult to feel thankful for your blessings. These foods can impact the immune system and cause illnesses.

Eating meals with friends and family can also help you appreciate your relationship with food. Eating together can create a sense of connection and camaraderie, making you more appreciative of the ones you love. When there is an opportunity to fellowship together, the food is appreciated differently. In addition, social eating can lead to a deeper conversation and a better understanding of each other.

When eating food, you can be reminded of the abundance that you have in your life. For example, eating something delicious can bring you joy and appreciation as you savor the flavors and taste, which allows you to explore how the food makes you feel.

Finally, you can use food to express your love and appreciation for others. Whether it's cooking a special meal for someone or bringing a treat to a gathering, food can be a powerful way to show gratitude for the people in your life.

The food you eat blesses you in numerous ways. It keeps you healthy and functioning to live an active life. It allows you to seek out your dreams and passions. Food brings us together with family and friends to foster an appreciation for the relationship and the time spent with them.

MINDFUL EATING: The practice of mindful eating has been researched and shows that as you slow down the pace of your meal, you notice how your body responds to the food you are eating. Slowing the pace of a meal gives you time to chew the food thoroughly before swallowing it.

Mindful eating can occur when you take a breath before eating and say a silent prayer of thanks. Food gratitude is one way of sharing the love for the foods that nourish our bodies and acknowledging the enjoyment that food brings us.

Expressing gratitude for your food lets you slowly become completely present while eating. Being present, you will chew your food well and have better digestion.

Counting Blessings Contribute to Healthy Living

When you take time in the mornings or evenings to write a gratitude letter, it helps you count the ways you are blessed. In writing the letter, positive wording helps relieve you of toxic emotions and supports your mental health. The letter allows you to focus on why you are grateful for life experiences and for the blessings from specific relationships that you have with others. In this way, you are less likely to contemplate your negative experiences. The letter can remain private, or you can send it to someone special to you. As the writer, you will benefit from the simple experience of writing the letter.

Your letter of gratitude becomes a reflection of the place within you that you have held like a flower bud that is now ready to bloom into a beautiful flower.

When you write a gratitude letter, you also lessen the stress that you might be experiencing. Stress is a mismatch between perceived demands and perceived ability to cope with requests. We are living in a world that is rapidly developing and need to learn how to manage stress.

Many changes in the world require quick adaptations and the ability to cope with uncertainties. The inability to adapt to the changes and delays can cause stress which can be hazardous to your well-being. Psychological stress can occur in the body with a physical cause. The gratitude letter can be an effective way of handling stressful situations. The letter serves as an outlet when needed for this type of stress and allows you to handle it better.

Gratefulness is a psychological force that can move you from a feeling of being overwhelmed to one of a feeling of being in control of your mental state. There is evidence that gratitude may have a lasting effect on the brain. Although not conclusive, the findings inform that practicing gratitude may help train the brain to be more sensitive to the experience of gratitude, which could lead to improved mental health. "Gratitude is good medicine," says Robert Emmons, Ph.D., a professor of psychology at the University of California, Davis, and the author of the *Little Book of Gratitude*.

EXAMPLE OF GRATITUDE LETTER

Dear Gratitude:

Thank you for reminding me of the good in my life, the good that resides in me, in others, and in the world. You have been a constant companion whispering words of encouragement and pointing out the beauty that surrounds me. Miracles abound small and large in your presence. I love the way you open my awareness of the beauty of a flower, the symmetry of a tall tree, or the appreciation of the comments of a loved one or stranger. You are always welcome in my life. I feel so much better when I notice your presence.

Writing the letter helps you appreciate life experiences and gives you a shift from negative thoughts and feelings to positive thoughts and feelings. Take a moment and write a gratitude letter.

"You must live in the present, launch yourself on every wave, find your eternity in each moment."

Henry David Thoreau

Chapter 4

WELL-BEING

The Other Side of Healthy Living

A focus on your well-being can often be neglected as you engage in your daily activities.

You may be focused on how others are doing but neglect yourself. As a result of this neglect, you may fail to notice what is happening to you when faced with a challenge or events which cause you to feel overwhelmed. In those moments, you might find yourself withdrawn or becoming angry. You realize that you were able to handle challenges before, but not now. In moments like these, you realize that you may need to place more of a focus on yourself and begin taking care of your mental health and well-being.

The experience of health, happiness, and prosperity defines the term well-being. It includes having good mental health, high life satisfaction, a sense of meaning or purpose, and managing stress. Well-being, in simple terms, is "just feeling good."

There is something that you can do to acquire the "just feel good" state. You can use gratitude to pull yourself up. Appreciation influences the brain and is linked to life satisfaction and improved well-being.

A 2019 study by Chinese Researchers found an initial neural basis relating gratitude to life satisfaction. The brains of the participants were influenced by how much appreciation they showed.

There are numerous ways and reasons for gratitude's improvement in your mental health. It starts with bringing self-value to yourself and others who feel valued in your life. As a result, there can be a decrease in anxiety, trauma, and stress and an increase in motivation, productivity, achievement, and self-worth.

If you are experiencing negative habits, gratitude can minimize those, as well as patterns of thinking and feeling. Gratitude improves joy, appreciation, kindness, generosity, and other positive expressions and behaviors. When you express gratitude as a habit, negative habit patterns of thinking and feeling, which often cause depression, panic, and fear, are minimized. Like a shower on a rainy day, gratitude can wash away concerns, worries, and self-doubt.

Do you remember when you were a child with an imagination that took you to faraway places and introduced you to magical characters? Well, gratitude can rekindle your inner childhood wonder. Additionally, feelings that are routinely expressed for nature, love, and connections bring out the inner child. This inner child is nonjudgmental and has a view of the positive side of life.

Embracing your inner child's wonder for the small things in life can motivate you to learn, grow, and improve or adapt to complex challenges and circumstances.

So, when expressing an abundance of good from gratitude, be prepared for much good in return. This will occur when you establish a daily gratitude practice. For example, you can start your day by being grateful for waking up, feeling refreshed, or for someone you love.

"The human heart has hidden treasures."

Bronte'

What are those treasures hidden in the human heart that Bronte speaks of? Might one of them be gratitude, thankfulness, or appreciation?

Our lives are full of reasons to feel thankful. There are times when we need to pause and remember to notice them. The frequent pauses with intentional focus will help you notice those reasons. When you start to use science-based techniques of gratitude consistently, good things begin to happen.

When you enhance your well-being, there is an immediate improvement in how you feel. From emotional wellness, good feelings can occur. Recognition that well-being emanates from thoughts, actions, and experiences helps you to monitor them and strive to keep the three of them in balance.

When you have a positive frame of mind, there is greater emotional well-being.

There are areas of well-being that should be acknowledged and embraced in your life. They are physical well-being, the ability to improve the functioning of your body through healthy living and good exercise habits. Next is social well-being, defined as the ability to communicate, develop meaningful relationships with others, and maintain a support network that helps you overcome loneliness.

Community well-being is the sense of engagement that you have with the area you live in. It's the ability to actively participate in a thriving community, culture, and environment.

Financial wellbeing involves all areas of well-being pertaining to your finances. This includes knowledge and skills in financial planning and management of expenses.

Workplace well-being is the ability to pursue your interests, values, and life purpose. It is gaining meaning, happiness, and enrichment professionally.

Spiritual well-being is having a sense of purpose or meaning and having a feeling of being connected to a higher power.

It takes time and effort to establish well-being skills. You will have to create a realistic plan, adhere to it, and take small daily actions. The ability to carry out your plan will enhance your life as you practice gratitude. These areas will strengthen your ability to utilize stress management, relaxation techniques, being resilient, boosting self-love, and generating emotions that lead to good feelings.

The feeling of having control of your life will help with the development of resilience. With resilience, you will focus on what you can do instead of thinking of yourself as a victim. Gratitude is one of the attributes that resilient individuals have because it allows them to face difficult situations and circumstances. When difficult situations occur, they believe that they are in control and regularly practicing gratitude helps with quicker recovery time from difficulties.

The mindset of resilient individuals gives them the attitude that they can make changes in the situations that are before them. It is not easy, however, to move from a place of negativity to one of gratefulness. The reason for this is simply that individuals are more familiar with and focus on the obstacles holding them back instead of the support that helps them to succeed.

The research of two academic psychologists, Shai Davidai and Thomas Gilovich found that individuals are often focused on immediate obstacles in front of them because of the need for immediate removal. The things that are supporting and sustaining them are not noticed. However, the practice of gratitude has many benefits affecting your well-being. The benefits include improved sleep, fewer health problems, fewer depressive symptoms, improved relationships, improved self-esteem, increased mental strength and resilience, improved positive action toward the fulfillment of goals, and improved ability to understand and share feelings with others.

The benefits of gratitude can bring change to your attitude and perspective, allowing you to shift from seeing only obstacles in life to appreciating what is good. Opening and extending this perspective, allows the world to make it easier for you to transition to being grateful for blessings.

Bob Proctor, an expert on gratitude, suggests a daily gratitude list consisting of three steps. Step one is to identify 10 things, people, and circumstances that you appreciate. Step two is to be quiet for 5 minutes and ask for guidance for the day. And Step three is to send love to three people who are bothering you. This practice is easy to complete. It can be carried out at the end of the day to acknowledge what happened during the day.

Practicing gratitude is beyond simply thinking about it. Regular practice includes acknowledging your gratitude to the people and support that elevate and assist you every day. It also involves realizing your uniqueness of you and the appreciation for self-value.

Your well-being gives you the courage and opportunity to have a pleasant life. Add gratefulness to your daily activities and see what a difference it makes in the way you feel.

Dan Millman said in a quote "Developing your well-being is a lifelong endeavor, but it is indeed worth it. You do not have to control your thoughts; you must stop letting them control you. "

Take pride in who you are and find ways to be the best you can be. Your well-being depends on it.

"Keeping your body healthy is an expression of Gratitude to the whole cosmos, the trees, the Clouds, everything."

Thich Nhat Hanh

Chapter 5

SELF-GRATITUDE

Appreciating Who You Are

Your day starts with getting dressed for work, getting the kids breakfast, getting them ready for school, and dropping them off. Next, you quickly stop at the post office to mail letters and then head to the office. Or you have only yourself to take care of and have a routine that you carry out every day. The many activities that you complete should make you feel good about their completion and thankful that you could do them. Congratulations on all that you have done in a short span of time.

Self-gratitude is defined as a thankfulness practice that affirms things about yourself that you appreciate. It is just as important as the practice of regular gratitude. There are numerous benefits attached to self-gratitude. These include lower stress, improved self-esteem, better days, and enjoyment of who you are as a person. It allows you to tap into your authentic self.

However, you may encounter negativity in your daily life and it affects you so that it becomes a dominant voice, coloring what is true and affecting how you feel about yourself. The negative voices inform you to turn a critical lens on yourself and point out as many flaws about what you don't like and chip away at your self-confidence and self-esteem. Negative self-talk is toxic and can even limit your dreams and ambitions. This toxicity causes misconceptions of situations and makes you jump to conclusions that are not based on the reality of a problem. Rather than examining facts, you end up looking at illusions.

Negative self-talk can be habitual and outside of your awareness. The opposite of negative self-talk is a self-gratitude dialogue that can help you accomplish your goals and dreams. It can challenge you to take up new adventures and reach new heights by setting new ones.

The ways that you can begin to eliminate negative self-talk is found in your ability to be an observer of your inner dialogue. Do not judge the conversation as it surfaces in your mind but observe its presence. Be conscious of the talk, where it occurs, and who you think of when the self-talk happens. The self-talk will quiet down and eventually disappear if you shift your focus from it.

When you can control self-criticism and self-doubt, you will find that you will have more compassion for yourself, recognizing that you have self-care and self-love for yourself the same way you care for family and friends. You come to understand that you have a purpose for living, that you have the power to grow, and seek the many possibilities that are waiting for you.

When focusing on self-gratitude, you can come to a place of realizing that you can contribute to the world with your gifts and talents. You also recognize that you are okay just the way you are in the present moment.

There is healing and motivating power in self-gratitude. Although there will be challenges and difficulties, choose self-gratitude to help you handle both.

Self-gratitude enables you to conquer self-doubt and not be discouraged or have a daunting opinion of yourself. It challenges fear and helps you reframe your thinking about what you are facing, giving you the courage to develop strategies for moving forward.

Positive self-talk or talk that is uplifting and encouraging affects your self-esteem or the positive or negative evaluation you have about yourself. It is the perceptions and interpretations of the world around you that affect your picture of yourself and your environment. Your self-esteem is high if you have high satisfaction with life. Low self-esteem is indicated when there is a low level of satisfaction. Researcher, Ozkan, stated that you can handle stress and establish social and close relationships if you have high self-esteem. You will have vitality and enjoyment in your life.

He further states if you have low self-esteem, your stamina, and enjoyment of life are affected. You will have less confidence and feelings of worthlessness or feel inadequate about your successes and skills. Empirical studies have shown if you are grateful, you have the inclination to have higher levels of self-esteem.

When you practice self-gratitude, you will embrace who you are, your traits, skills, talents, knowledge, style, choices, and physical self.

There is often a lot of pressure to be like everyone else. However, being different and trying new things can be enjoyable and refreshing. When it comes to being your authentic self, there is nothing wrong with taking risks. Being different is a form of self-expression allowing you to have freedom from the script written by others for you.

When you show yourself increased gratitude, it helps you to appreciate who you are and your uniqueness. When you appreciate yourself, you won't try to be perfect, punish yourself, pass up opportunities, be afraid of yourself, or depend on others for their approval. Remember it is often conditioning that leads you to believe that it is not in your best interest to think, feel, or have the experiences you are having. However, when you become aware of the full range of your potential and enjoy all that the potential has to offer, appreciation and compassion for who you are will expand.

Understand that it takes responsibility to be the person you have always wanted to be. Now, take the responsibility of being your own best friend, learning to give unconditional love and acceptance to yourself and others. If any part of yourself is excluded the love given will be conditional. Therefore, make the love unconditional and find that life transformation takes place.

There are many ways to practice self-gratitude. Using daily affirmations is one way. Writing statements that are true about yourself can make you feel good. These affirmations focus on the good about you and your contributions to the world. Affirmations can change your thinking about yourself and strengthen your confidence.

The affirmations below are examples of some that you might use.

Self-Gratitude Affirmations:

I am confident about how I speak my truth when speaking to others.

I am knowledgeable and use my knowledge wisely when interacting with others.

I expect good things to happen to me when I engage and dialogue with others in my daily life.

I love and appreciate who I am as a person.

I feel good about myself and what I can do when completing goals.

I am loving, caring, compassionate, kind, gentle, patient and understanding.

I love who I am and embrace all that I can be.

I look in the mirror and say to myself, I love you.

Along with affirmations, try to find new things to notice about yourself as you engage in your daily activities. When you begin to look for new things about yourself, you will find no limit to them.

Remember to write down what you notice for a few weeks and discover your uniqueness. Recognize and acknowledge your strengths and celebrate them. Some of the things you might celebrate include appreciating yourself for every thought and act of kindness, thinking of at least one loving thing you do for yourself each day, and saying "thank you" to yourself when you do something kind. And, getting comfortable with telling yourself, "I love you."

There is beauty and power in self-gratitude, which allows you to appreciate who you are in the present moment. It gives you permission to embrace your uniqueness. Regular practice of self-gratitude can be very rewarding personally and in relationships with others. When you appreciate yourself, and give yourself love and respect, then you can share all that you are with those you love and others. Your radiance is noticed by those who have the chance to be in your presence. A good feeling is felt by others who experience the radiance and warmth that comes from you.

Take a moment and set the book down and focus on why you appreciate yourself. What thoughts come to mind about you? How would you describe yourself? How do you feel about the person you have become? Take pen to paper and write for 10 minutes focusing on you. What did you discover about yourself?

Author Cheri Huber says "The only difference between the life you are living and the life you want to live is the feeling of being appreciated, loved, and accepted unconditionally. When experiencing self-gratitude, you will find that unconditional love and acceptance become part of your life. There is no better time than now to embrace it."

QUOTES

"Do we dare be ourselves? That is the question that counts." Pablo Casals

"No matter what happens to you, there is a positive outcome that awaits. There's a lesson and there is growth to be had from everything."

Kaya Wittenburg

"Your vision will become clear only when you investigate your own heart. Who looks outside, dreams. Who looks inside, awakes."

Carl Jung

"When you take care of yourself, you are a better person for others. When you feel good about yourself, you treat others better."

Solange

Chapter 6

GRATITUDE & RELATIONSHIPS

The More You Give, the More You Get

When you think of gratitude and relationships, you may think of romantic relationships. However, there is so much more to relationships to be considered when you practice gratitude.

A relationship is defined as being connected to another person or the way you regard and behave toward each other. Becoming aware of how relationships in your life mirror the one you have with yourself is key to understanding and nourishing those you have with others.

To begin the journey of being grateful, you start with yourself. Then, while practicing self-gratitude, a foundation is created that allows you to show gratitude and compassion to others. Your kindness, gentleness, patience, and understanding are a gift that others will benefit from because of the love you have for yourself. According to Nathaniel Brandon, a therapist and lecturer, high self-esteem rests on six pillars. These include living consciously, accepting yourself, taking responsibility for individual actions, being self-assertive, living with purpose, and having personal integrity. It is from these pillars that a love of yourself can develop, and stronger relationships can be built.

Having the ability to use self-control and gratitude behaviors are interrelated. High levels of self-control elicit gratitude, while low levels of self-control do the opposite. Less gratitude is expressed when there is a low level of self-control. Individuals who experience increased gratitude appear to be more satisfied with life and have greater happiness and commitment in their relationships.

Personal and relational well-being is influenced by gratitude. For example, after receiving benefits from others, people feel more grateful when the person giving the gifts acts in a way that is perceived as thoughtful and responsive to their needs.

An additional way to practice unique self-care and gratitude is found in the practice of cradling work. This practice was described by Angeles Aruen, who is a cultural anthropologist. According to Aruen, this is a practice of self-acknowledgment found in parts of Africa and Oceanic societies. Cradling work acknowledges oneself and the connection to what is accurate, sound, and beautiful about the self. There are four parts to the practice of cradling work.

First, it begins with lying on the floor and placing both hands over the heart.

In silence, one proceeds to:

Acknowledge the character qualities that one appreciates about oneself.

Next, acknowledge one's strengths and talents.

Finally, recognize the contributions one has made in the past and the present.

Acknowledge the love one has given and is giving, and the loved one who received and is receiving.

Cradling work as a practice should be performed three times a day, morning, afternoon, and night to be of benefit.

This practice gives you an opportunity to form an awareness of who you are. It helps to form a relationship with the self that can be carried over to developing relationships with others. A caring and loving attitude begins to manifest.

A gratitude disposition helps to create immeasurable connections in relationships, inspiring you toward a shared and meaningful purpose. Numerous situations benefit from an expression of gratitude. Therefore, building relational connections can be practiced in a variety of ways. For example, you take time to reduce your busy schedule and visit with a friend or go for a walk in a park and appreciate the scenery of Nature with a family member or you take time to call a friend that you have not heard from in awhile to let them know that you missed your connection with them.

Or you schedule a time daily or once a week to call a friend or family member to let them know you care about them and want to know how they are doing.

Examples of situations that merit an expression of gratitude might include love for the family, feelings of belonging with others you value in your life, celebrating the achievements of others, or appreciation for being acknowledged by others for what you have done for them.

When relationships are formed, it is wise to be a good listener. You listen to the ideas and experiences of the person you are with and learn their strengths, which can enhance your relationship. As an active listener, you will also recognize and appreciate their efforts and acknowledge the abilities and perspectives that they share with you. Therefore, taking time to listen lets them know that you are interested in them as a person and place value on who they are.

Remember, everyone can express gratitude. However, for some individuals, this may not happen spontaneously. Strength in the expression of gratitude is developed through practice, and practice helps to open channels that allow for openness with each other.

A grateful disposition promotes experiences of gratitude and is linked to greater well-being. Several of the well-being rewards of expressed gratitude are those of being more satisfied in life, being more optimistic, and being less depressed. As a result, there is less rumination about negative experiences. Feeling grateful encourages and motivates people to help others and, in turn, feel good about themselves.

When it comes to strengthening relationships, gratitude is at the forefront of making it happen. Research shows that expressing gratitude for the people you care about improves the relationship for both of you by bringing you closer to each other and helping to sustain the relationship.

The expression of gratitude shows that you care by acknowledging a trait in the other person. It is a powerful way of demonstrating affection and bringing a measure of closeness to the relationship.

A study of 75 years by Robert Waldinger on adult development sites shows how relationships are the most significant predictor of health and happiness.

Along with being a predictor of health and happiness, strong relationships can help us cope with stress, reduce the risk of illness, and even boost the immune system.

Our relationships help us feel connected to each other and provide a sense of purpose, bringing joy, peace, and meaning to our lives.

A quote by Jane Seymour beautifully expresses the reason for having positive relationships.

She says: "I know that the purpose of life is to understand and be in the present moment with the people you love. It's just that simple."

Relationship Quotes:

"It is not our purpose to become each other; it is to recognize each other, to learn to see each other, and to honor those we love for who they are."

Hermann Hesse

"Being deeply loved by someone gives you strength while loving someone deeply gives you courage."

Lao Tzu

"I have learned that people will forget what you said, people will forget what you did, but people will never forget how you made them feel."

Maya Angelou

"The meeting of two personalities is like the contact of two chemical substances: if there is any reaction both are transformed."

Carl Gustav Jung

Chapter 7

JOURNALING & GRATITUDE

Rethinking In a Creative Way

Many events and experiences call one's attention to them, increasing anxiety and stress. In trying to sort out all the noise in your head, you focus on what's important. However, you have a difficult time doing so.

The thoughts attached to those mental space grabbers continue to swirl in your mind. Family concerns, relationship with your spouse, questions about whether you are spending enough time together. You question whether you are doing things that strengthen your relationship with your family, loved ones, and yourself.

What happens when you are also experiencing job issues? For example, a promotion is waiting for you depending on your performance review. Have you completed all the job requirements at or above a satisfactory level?

Your continual thoughts of spousal relationship, parental needs, parenting a child, and job review have placed you on mental overload. So, what are you to do?

Where can you find relief from the stress that is bubbling over? Is there relief to be found? The answer is yes to your question. The practice of gratitude journaling can help you with stressful and challenging situations. Focusing on gratefulness helps maintain a proper perspective and lessens the time that distress finds a home in your life.

Webster's Dictionary describes journaling as a record of experiences, ideas, or reflections kept for private use.

The use of journals has taken place over a long period of time. It is said that journal writing is as old as the art of writing itself. The origins of the modern journal occurred in fifteenth-century Italy, where diaries/journals were used for accounting. After that, the focus slowly shifted from recording public life to reflecting a recording of private life.

The ideas for inventions and observations were recorded by Leonardo Da Vinci in journals that were made up of 5,000 pages. Famous people like Charles Darwin, Marie Curie, Thomas Jefferson, and Albert Einstein kept journals they used to record their thoughts. Benjamin Franklin wrote in his morning journal using the prompt, "What good shall I do this day." And in the evening, he used the prompt, "What good have I done today?" Oprah Winfrey used a journal for many years and contributed much of her success to journaling. The journal has been a successful tool for many great men and women.

The Center for Journal Therapy was established in 1985 by Kathleen Adams, a Psychotherapist in Colorado. Adams became the founder/director of the Center and began teaching journal workshops. The workshops were developed to give the public tools that could be used for self-discovery, life enhancement, and creative expression. Workshops are held throughout the year.

The medical and therapeutic communities began to take a closer look at journal writing as a nonmedical method for wellness because of the Pennebaker Studies published in 1997. His studies revealed that expressive writing could improve health.

Many adults have found journaling beneficial for mental, emotional, and spiritual illumination.

The power of journaling for clarification of experiences is numerous. First, it is a method of writing about your thoughts and feelings and gaining an understanding of them by viewing them in writing. Writing in a journal can also bring emotions to the surface and allow for mental clarity and focus. Finally, it helps you navigate beyond entrenched negative thoughts and feelings.

Journaling can also help sharpen your memory and improve your cognitive ability. So, let's get started and look at ways that one or several journals can be used to help you find the gift that gratitude has to offer through the medium of journaling. Using a journal will allow you to move thoughts that are stressing you out by giving you a chance to write about them.

As a result of writing your thoughts, you empty your mental vault and then have an opportunity to examine what you found in there. Seeing your thoughts in writing allows you to choose what is of value to you and release any thoughts that do not serve you well.

There are several types of journals that you might use to record your internal thoughts. Several are listed for your review.

The Gratitude Journal

The gratitude journal will enable you to write about all the things you find grateful in your life.

You can write about small things that you are thankful for as well as the more important things that enter your life or write about the people you are grateful for and experiences you encounter.

While writing in this journal, you will come to appreciate the gifts of life and those you may think of as a bag of rocks. The Persian poet, Rumi living in the 13th Century, wrote, "Gratitude should be worn like a clock, and it will feed every corner of your life." When you begin using a gratitude journal, you will discover that the small and simple things in life support you on your life journey positively.

A journal might require some organizing. You might begin by writing the date and beginning time, before starting to write about your day. If you can't think of a place to start, a journal prompt might help in getting you started with your writing. A journal prompt is a statement or question that helps you to start writing. It is useful when you have a writing block or need help with what to write. Here are some prompts for you to consider:

I am joyful…

My day went well because…

I am grateful for my family because…

I am thankful for wonderful relationships because…

When I think of my job, I am pleased because…

I am thankful for the negatives in my life because…

I feel most peaceful because…

My heart is feeling grateful today because…

Even when things aren't going well, try to find something within the situation or experience to be thankful for and take a deep breath to relax your body and mind. If you are having difficulty with an individual, see the humanity in them and find something about them to be grateful for.

Do not leave yourself out; think and write about self-gratitude. In what ways are you thankful for who you are as a person, as a friend, family member, lover, or neighbor?

The gratitude journal is one of the most potent journals because it helps you view your life experiences from a different perspective. This journal is all about you and who you are as a person. There are many hidden gems that you will discover about yourself. The gratitude journal has been highlighted and shown to benefit significantly from capturing your thoughts about life experiences.

There are several other types of journals that you can incorporate into your writing experiences. These will extend your shift toward life experiences as you encounter them. The next journal will allow you to tap into your creative side if you like to draw or sketch.

ART JOURNAL

The Art Journal is a creative way to solve problems and reduce stress. It is a form of personal expression without the pressure of perfection while working in your journal.

Developing an art journal can be a pleasant experience because you can use it to capture experiences you want to remember. Unlike when utilizing a camera, you become an intimate part of the creative process.

Writing and drawing can go together when you are working in this journal. A combination of the two will add an impressive feature to the page due to the art and colors you use when you choose to incorporate the mediums of crayons, chalk, watercolors, pens, and colored pencils. You will find that using your thoughts and feelings as a guide will inspire you to write, draw, and express your emotions while relieving stress.

Some art journals may resemble scrapbooks, sketchbooks, or diaries. Since there are no rules for what your art journal should look like, your creative expression is all that matters. You will find that the process helps you to relax and think of the positives in your life. Gratitude finds a place in your thoughts and gives you the gift of feeling better about yourself and others.

INSPIRATIONAL JOURNAL

This journal reminds you of how others used words to uplift and move their thoughts to a place of inspiration. To begin this journal, you will need to find and collect quotes that you can write in your journal or type quotes and paste them in place. After reading and logging the quote, write how you felt while reading it and your thoughts after reading it. Being inspired by the quotes of others should pique your interest in writing your own as a creative way of expressing who you are and your interpretation of your world.

The inspirational quotes below are some of my favorites.

"When I let go of what I am, I become what I might be." Lao Tzu

"Appreciate where you are and enjoy the journey as you work toward where you are going."

Jenna Ortega

"Understand the laws of creation and awaken your surface to the realization that you are truly loved. After all, understanding is simply loving, and loving is the expression of self, you." Mary

"Wake at dawn with a winged heart and give thanks for another day of loving." Kahlil Gibran

"Something opens our wings. Something makes boredom and hurt disappear. Someone fills the cup in front of us. We taste only sacredness." Rumi

"Life is full of beauty. Notice it. Notice the bumble bee, the small child, and the smiling faces. Smell the rain and feel the wind. Live your life to the fullest potential, and fight for your dreams." Ashley Smith

The inspiring words of others will cause you to have a different perspective about people, places, and things. Inspirational quotes can be found in books; however, you can also listen in on conversations and hear someone repeat their favorite quote.

WHEN TO JOURNAL

One of the best times to journal is in the early morning before the start of your day. This can set the tone for your day because of the elevation of your mood. The evening hours can be used to reflect on daily activities or explore how well you managed your everyday experiences.

Having a comfortable or convenient place to do your journaling can help set the mood for your writing expressions. The space you decide to use for journaling can be an area you have set aside just for this activity. A park bench setting in nature can be a calm and peaceful place to journal in the afternoon.

When you start journaling, take small steps by writing about one or two things you are grateful for each day of the month. Your gratitude can flow when you become comfortable with the process.

And finally, take time to make Nature a part of your life, as it has a variety of journal themes for you to write about, draw, or sketch. There are no limits to what you will encounter in Nature, so be prepared to choose between what you will capture and include in your journal.

JOURNAL MATERIAL

You can start your journal journey with a notebook, diary, or just sheets of paper stapled together. A variety of journal materials will allow you to have more of an extraordinary creative experience. Here are some ideas to get you started on your journey.

Select plain or decorative journals.

Collect a set of pens

Colored pen set

Pencils

Colored pencils

Pencil sharpener

Watercolors

Sticky notes to write ideas on

Stickers of choice

Photos taken with a camera.

Pictures cut from magazines.

Personal sketches

Gratitude quote books

Inspirational quote books

Try being creative and make your own journal to capture your thoughts and feelings. This process captures your energy and becomes part of you.

Use cardboard or food boxes to make a junk journal using scraps of paper or recycled material. This can be creative and fun. The junk journal can be a wonderful place to record your thoughts, dreams, and project ideas and expression of gratitude.

Journaling is a form of self-therapy that allows you to show your inner thoughts about your life experiences and accept them as you acknowledge what those experiences are by writing about them in unique ways.

There is always an opportunity to view what you have written and see the internal growth that you have made. Growth in learning how to release stressful situations, how to honor the good, and most importantly how to embrace who you are as a person. You start to become the person you want to be and begin to take control of your life with confidence and gratitude. The journaling process releases inspiration and strengthens you.

Take a moment to enjoy these journal quotes:

"Your journal is like your best friend; you don't have to pretend with it, you can be honest and write exactly how you feel." Bukola Ogunwale

"If you do not breathe through writing, if you do not cry out in writing, or sing in writing, then don't write, because our culture has no use for it."

Anais Nin

"Journaling helps you to remember how strong you truly are within yourself." Asad Meah

"Journaling helps you express all that is good in your life, capture the good, and save it in the vaults of memory."

Theresa M. Ross

"Journaling is like a camera; it captures your thoughts and allows you to see how magnificent you are."

Theresa M. Ross

"Look for the golden nuggets among the rocks while journaling and be grateful that you found them."

Theresa M. Ross

Chapter 8

COLORS INFLUENCE GRATITUDE

The Power of Color Hues

Take a moment to look around the setting that you are in and identify the colors that you see. These colors are those that you were drawn to because of the way they made you feel.

Colors play a significant role in our lives. They impact our moods, inspire decision-making, and influence what we think. The colors we see are compelling in how they affect our lives.

You might notice a shift in your attitude when encountering a particular color. The color may have caused a feeling of nostalgia, and you may have attributed the experience to a typical human response. There is a deeper meaning to the experience.

However, the cause is far more complex. According to color psychology, a great deal of human behavior is dictated by color. Therefore, an understanding of the possibilities of the effect of color determines how we perceive the world of color.

In 1704, Isaac Newton's book Opticks described the color wheel, showing how each color is determined by a different wavelength of light. Newton's work assisted in color being understood in scientific terms. He realized white light has many colors within it when a prism is placed in sunlight and a rainbow can be viewed on the other side of the prism.

Johanna Wolfgang Goethe was the first person to study the physiological effects of color systematically. He published *The Color Theory* in 1810 to describe his findings. Goethe divided the colors into two groups. One group (red, orange, and yellow) included colors he defined as those that caused happiness. The second group had (green, blue, and yellow) colors that caused sadness. Goethe found that colors can cause both happiness and sadness.

Ancient practitioners of color therapy and modern researchers have demonstrated that color can touch and bring balance to an individual on a physical, emotional, mental, and spiritual level. Some colors can be warm, some are cool, and others soothe and stimulate the observer.

Most individuals experience color through vision as they enjoy the array of colors in their view. However, there are some individuals who not only see colors but also feel colors. If an individual feels color, they may experience it as a warm or comforting feeling when they see red, orange, or yellow.

The colors you choose to wear and surround yourself with influence your mood, body, and mind. The effect of the colors may occur in subtle as well as not-so-subtle ways.

Modern research confirms that colors can influence your thoughts and behavior. It is known that different colors activate specific areas of the brain and can trigger certain emotions and behaviors. Color is a powerful form of communication.

Let's look at the characteristics of several colors and their effect on mood, well-being, and health in general.

Red has been examined more than any other color in health performance and psychology. Red is linked to excitement, dominance, passion, anger, and aggression. According to research studies, red clothing can raise your heart rate and increase your strength because it can cause you to react quickly and with more force.

When it comes to a calming effect and an increase in focus and creativity, lighter shades of blue are recommended; blue shades can remind you of the ocean or the sky and bring about relaxation and peace. It has a significant impact on your emotions and thoughts as well.

Green is rated as the most pleasant of colors, except for blue. Although Goethe placed green under the category of sadness, further research discovered that green could affect you in many ways. Surround yourself with green to experience peace and boost your positivity. Green is a restful color of balance, harmony, refreshment, rest, and restoration.

For an expression of joy and positivity, select yellow. This color is a reminder of the warmth of the sun or a sunny day. Clinical studies revealed that yellow lights caused feelings of happiness and reduced negative emotions such as anger and depression; if you want to have an uplifting day wear yellow clothing.

Rudolf Steiner, an Austrian philosopher, developed a color philosophy that gives a schedule for wearing colors in clothing and jewelry. A color is chosen for each day of the week. The key is wearing or surrounding yourself with the color chosen for the day.

Monday is a day to wear purple, Tuesday pink, Wednesday yellow, Thursday orange or brown, Friday green, Saturday blue, and Sunday white. According to this philosophy, colors create a sense of balance, rhythm, and order.

Every color can affect you physically, emotionally, mentally, and spiritually. Since colors come in a variety of tones, brightness, shades, and tints, the characteristics of the color can have different effects on the mood and emotions of an individual.

Exploring how color influences gratitude is a relevant topic since it fits into the realm of positive psychology.

According to psychology, colors play an essential role in life and individuals often associate different colors with different emotions.

However, being grateful has a much deeper meaning because it is a feeling, a positive emotion, and has a purpose. The feeling of gratitude can be expressed with colors, mainly pink. This color has an aura of elegance and grace about it. There is a radiance of romance and sweetness. The variation of dark pink is often used to represent gratitude and appreciation.

Individuals have purchased red roses to show their love and passion. In many ways, the red color of the roses resembles a dark pink pigment and carries with it the feeling of gratitude.

If you want to express your gratitude to someone, why not use pink paper to write a note? Or use a pen or marker with pink ink to write your message. The use of color will enhance the effects of your actions.

When you explore various colors and their meaning regarding emotions and gratitude, other regions of your life are affected. Let's look at the type of birthstone jewelry you wear.

BIRTHSTONES AND THEIR MEANING

Most people wear their birthstone jewelry because they think of the beauty of it. However, birthstones are not only related to the month you are born in, but they have their own unique meaning. Because of the color of the birthstones, depending on your birth month, there will be some influence on your life.

January – Garnet comes in several shades. The most popular color is reddish brown. It can also be found in other colors, purple, pink, violet, brown, yellow, orange, and black. The birthstone was considered a great gift to represent friendship and trust. At other times, it could express purification, love, strength, intense feelings, and balance.

February – Amethyst (purple) is a birthstone that brings peace and tranquility to the wearer. It is stated that amethyst can strengthen the bond of love between two people. This color is associated with royalty and nobility. It represents sincerity, security, spirituality, and contentment.

March – Aquamarine (blue) youthfulness, hope, love, and encourages the making of new friends and relationships.

April – The diamond (transparent with no hue) is associated with love which makes it a perfect gift for a loved one. Diamonds are the most popular gemstone.

May – Emerald (green) This birthstone carries the essence of wisdom, faith, success in love, and domestic bliss. It is known for its brilliant, rich green color. It is also characterized as having healing abilities bringing spiritual rebirth and renewal to the wearer.

June – Pearl comes in many different colors. Classic white, pink, yellow, golden, black, and every shade. Black pearl is the most popular, and blue is the rarest. Pearl expresses success, happiness, and love.

July – Rubies' color can be a vibrant red to a purplish red. They are considered the king of gems and represent love, health, and wisdom,

August – Peridot (Olivine) is green, like an emerald. The gem of Peridot expresses strength and instills power and influence in the wearer.

September – Sapphire comes in various colors, including green, pink, white, and yellow. However, it is associated with blue hues most often. The purity of sapphire reveals heavenly grace and embodies the characteristics of loyalty, trust, and faithfulness.

October – Opal can be found in red, orange, and yellow. Blue and green are considered fewer common colors. It is believed to bring happiness, healing, innocence, and hope.

November – Citrine can be found in light pastel and a reddish-orange color. It is believed to symbolize faithfulness and friendship.

December – Tanzanite can range in color from a rich blue to violet. This is a stone that is believed to connect a person to the spiritual realm. In addition, it is thought to keep the dignity and integrity of the wearer intact while transmitting peace of mind.

While examining the colors of the birthstones and their characteristics, you can observe their connection to the feeling of gratitude. Such words as friendship, trust, happiness, sincerity, love, wisdom, faithfulness, and peace of mind can be found as a part of the makeup of the birthstone.

CRYSTALS

Another fascinating area is the color of unique crystals and their relationship to gratitude. We begin with an understanding that to be grateful starts with appreciating all that is good in your life. So please do not overlook the little or small things, for they also count.

The crystal rose quartz is a great one for gratitude expression. It has a gentle vibration and will teach you to see the world with more love and compassion.

Amethyst can transmute negative energy into loving and calming energy. It is a popular crystal that can be used for gratitude. Carrying amethyst on your person can help focus the mind on positive thoughts.

Chrysocolla brings calmness and is often used to encourage gratefulness. Remembering past challenging experiences will help you to be grateful for the present moment. The gentle vibrations of the chrysocolla will assist you in seeing how far you have come. Your awareness of this will shift your feelings.

Malachite transforms the mindset and moves you to a place of thankfulness. It gives you the perspective that makes you more aware of things you take for granted.

You can try clear quartz crystal to see the positive side of any situation or challenge, it brings a confident feeling that everything will work out in your best interest. As a result, you become grateful for such confidence.

When you are feeling a need to be abundantly grateful, bring Aquamarine into your orbit. This crystal will bring clarity to any situation, show you how little things make you happy, and teach you to appreciate these little things.

Crystals, along with birthstones, have a powerful influence on our lives. The energy that both carry is transferred and affects our thought processes.

From a place of negativity, there is an upliftment to positivity and the words that connect to gratitude flow forth. Words like friendship, trust, love, wisdom, faithfulness, peace of mind, thankfulness, and gratitude become common.

Colors in birthstones, crystals, and everyday ordinary places and things have a profound effect on how we feel, and our perception of life experiences. When selecting colors, choose wisely because you want to be aware of what you express emotionally, physically, and spiritually.

Color Quotes

"Colors, like features, follow the changes of the emotions."

Pablo Picasso

"How I dress is the way I feel. If I'm wearing bright colors, I'm probably in a good mood."

Willie Cauley-Stein

"I try to apply colors like words that shape poems, like notes that shape music."

Joan Miro

Chapter 9

MINDFULNESS AND GRATITUDE

The Benefit of Being in the Moment

Mindfulness and gratitude are two powerful practices that can help bring peace and joy into your life. It involves being in the moment and focusing on your thoughts, feelings, and the present situation. As a result, you have an opportunity to recognize and appreciate life's beauty, even facing challenges.

In working with the practice of gratitude, it enables you to identify and enjoy all the blessings in your life. You learn to be grateful on a larger scale and a smaller one.

When you practice mindfulness and gratitude together, you can better understand yourself, your relationships, and the world around you.

An awareness of your thoughts and feelings can help you recognize and appreciate the positive in your life and be grateful for your blessings. Practicing gratitude opens you to the wonders of life and brings joy to enjoy the simple moments that your experiences present to you.

Your practice of mindfulness and gratitude can cultivate a greater sense of peace, joy, and contentment. It can bring an abundance of connections to us and the world around us. There can be more openness to giving and receiving love. We can have increased mindfulness about our choices and actions. It can cause greater compassion and kindness to us and others.

Mindfulness practice involves learning to relax, staying present without judging, and remaining open and mentally flexible. It is giving attention to the contents of a given moment. It is a practice of giving attention carefully and on purpose. When you develop a daily practice of meditation, a disciplined routine takes place.

To teach yourself how to be in the present moment, you need to pay attention purposefully. As you become comfortable with being mindful through meditation, you will find that you become relaxed and aware.

The emphasis when practicing mindfulness is on being; you have nothing to do. Mindfulness relies on observing your thoughts while focusing on your breath. Freedom comes from accepting what is happening in your mind or around you. Distractions are to be witnessed, as this is the essence of mindfulness practice.

When you mindfully approach life, you meet and connect with each experience you encounter through the present moment. If practiced daily, mindfulness becomes a way of living as it is grounded in your life through meditation.

You may be thinking about whether mindfulness works. However, the only way for you to know if it does or not is to give it a try. And notice what happens because of your effort.

Recent research has affirmed that mindfulness has excellent benefits when practiced daily. In addition, it has been linked to both health and healing.

According to Lyn Freeman, "Mindfulness is a non-concentrative technique where an individual opens their consciousness to observe in a non-judgmental way their thoughts and mental activities. With mindfulness, you are empowered to be present at any given moment."

As mentioned earlier, mindfulness is developed through meditation. In this meditation practice, there are direct experiences of attention and awareness centered on thoughts and all other aspects of affairs in the present moment. Therefore, a commitment must be made to being mindful and paying attention to purpose in daily life.

Although Buddhists have practiced meditation for 2,500 years, mindfulness is not connected to religious or spiritual traditions. Therefore, a particular belief system and spiritual or religious views are not required to practice it. As you practice mindfulness, identification patterns with your experiences will soften, and you will find greater peace and harmony with life. Gratitude begins entering your inner being and gaining expression in your outer environment because mindfulness accurately reflects all we possess. So much of life is missed due to misinformed perceptions and habitual ways of acting, feeling, and thinking.

The success of a meditation practice requires both internal and external conditions to be related to the procedure. The internal conditions are based on several crucial factors. The first factor is a positive attitude, whereby you take the approach of not knowing everything. Secondly, you must be interested in gaining a greater understanding of yourself and your life as it manifests. Thirdly, you must be willing to accept unpleasant and challenging moments. Fourth, you must develop confidence in handling and managing your thoughts, feelings, and actions.

The practice of daily meditation requires that you identify a place for practice and establish a routine. There must be consistency which will help to create daily meditation habits. The time for meditating is up to you. You might decide to practice meditation in the morning, which is preferable, or in the evening.

So, remember the following words as you decide to develop your practice. These are attitude, curiosity, motivation, determination, discipline, and belief in yourself. Each word embraces critical internal factors.

You will need to recognize the importance of internal factors which does not negate the fact that external factors also need to be identified in your practice. When doing so, it helps to build a strong foundation when you become aware of these factors. The foundation includes where you practice, when practice is done, the support of family, and the acquisition and careful use of tapes and readings. Also, be aware of things that might interfere with your practice. Try for a time when you will not be disturbed by other people or external demands. Be sure to have enough energy to practice and not be affected by sleepiness or drowsiness, which can interfere with your practice.

You may have to experiment to find the best place and time for meditation practice. When you have decided on the location and time, you will now want to decide on the practice program that is of interest to you.

There is both a formal and informal meditation approach. In traditional meditation, you will have a period when your meditation is your main activity. Formal meditation can be practiced once a day for at least thirty minutes. Informal practice is the use of mindfulness throughout the day as situations happen. Attention is given to the condition itself, or contact can be made with the problem by conscious breathing, connecting mind and body in the present moment.

You will need to encourage yourself to do formal mindfulness practice since there will be times when you do not feel like it. You may experience resistance, but be patient with yourself, encouraging and pushing forward with an attitude of conquering resistance and continuing to meditate.

Informal practice can be essential and helpful in reminding yourself to practice mindfulness throughout the day to be present in the moment.

The heart and mind receive training when you bring mindfulness into your life. So be ready to get energy, effort, and discipline into your practice.

Mindfulness Meditation Instructions
One of the easiest ways to practice mindful meditation is to follow your breath. Belly breath or diaphragmatic

breathing is the foundation of mindfulness practice. Belly breathing involves using your belly to guide air into your lungs rhythmically. This breathing differs from the typical breathing pattern of tight short breaths in the chest. When practicing breathing be sure to observe whether you are breathing from the chest area or the belly. There will be a distinct difference between the two.

To practice belly breaths:

1. Begin by finding a comfortable position, either sitting or lying down.
2. Next, close your eyes and take a few deep breaths.
3. Next, bring your awareness to your body and scan it from head to toe, noticing any sensations that arise.
4. Now bring your awareness to your breath, noticing the sensation of the breath as it enters and leaves your body.
5. Place one hand on the chest and the other on the belly button.
6. Breathe so your hand is on the belly button and is pushed out as you inhale to fill your lungs with air.
7. Your belly is pulled in as air leaves your lungs when you exhale.
8. The chest hand remains stationary as much as possible.
9. If your mind begins to wander or becomes distracted, observe the thought and feeling without judgment and gently bring your attention back to your breath.

10. Continue to observe your breath for several minutes.
11. Then, when you are ready, slowly open your eyes and take a few moments to reflect on the experience.

Developing your breathing may take some practice, but you should be able to master it over time.

One of the ways of recording your progress is to keep a journal that includes the number of minutes practiced and the questions that arise or problems that need attention. Practicing with others can be a powerful support system and encouragement when you feel challenged about your meditation practice.

Remember, mindfulness and gratitude go together because shifting the mind to what is happening now and observing thoughts and mental activity allows you to focus on family, friends, acquaintances, and things that you are grateful for in your life experiences.

Mindfulness Quotes

"Gratefulness and happiness begin with falling in love with yourself." Theresa M. Ross

"To know yourself as the Being underneath the thinker, the stillness underneath the mental noise, the love and joy underneath the pain, is freedom, salvation, enlightenment." Eckhart Tolle

Chapter 10

AFFIRMATIONS IMPACT GRATITUDE

Gratitude and affirmations are closely related because both involve recognizing and expressing positive emotions. Gratitude is a feeling of appreciation for the good things in life, while affirmations are positive statements used to encourage and uplift oneself. Both gratitude and affirmation can help to improve mental health, reduce stress, and increase resilience. Additionally, both can be used to recognize and appreciate the good things one has in life while helping to create a mindset of abundance and positivity.

Affirmations have been around for centuries, with some of the earliest references found in ancient East Indian and Chinese texts. These affirmations were used to help people focus on the positive and to help improve their physical, mental, and spiritual health.

The modern use of affirmations dates to the 19th Century when French philosopher Emile Coue developed the concept of autosuggestion. Coue believed that by repeating positive affirmations, one could reprogram one's subconscious mind and bring about positive changes in one's life. His ideas were later popularized by American New Thought movement leaders such as Napoleon Hill and Emmet Fox, who wrote extensively on the power of positive thinking. In the 1960s and 1970s, affirmations gained further popularity, thanks to the work of self-help authors such as Louise Hay, who wrote a best-selling book on the topic. Her work helped affirmations become a mainstream tool for personal development and self-improvement.

In recent years, affirmations have become increasingly popular, with many people using them daily to help them stay focused on achieving their goals. They have also been used in psychotherapy, with some therapists using them as part of cognitive behavioral therapy.

Affirmations can be defined as a way of putting forth intention for what you would like to create in your life. They are a fantastic way of giving strength in helping you to develop a pattern of gratitude. It would be best if you were intentional about the gratitude you wish to express. Take time to get quiet, still the mind, and center your consciousness deeply with yourself.

When you use an affirmation, know that it should be at once personal, positive, and stated in the present tense with emotion, understanding, and acceptance.

At once, personal means that the affirmation is phrased to be specifically related to you. For example, instead of saying, "May good health manifest for all people of the world," say, "I give thanks that good health is manifesting at once in my life.

Always personalize your affirmation by using "I." Using "I" makes it personal and centered on you. It is necessary to make sure that what you are affirming has a positive aspect.

You want to verbalize what you want instead of what you do not want. By doing so, you emphasize the positive pattern you want to experience. The language should be stated in the present tense to keep you current and attached to the affirmation immediately.

When you state in the present tense, you comment that something is happening in the moment, not in the future or imaginary time. The following phrases, such as "going to" or "trying," should be avoided. For example, the statement, "I accept that I am going to try and be happier." This statement is not happening in the present. Instead, it can be stated as, I give thanks that each day, I am experiencing greater happiness and expressing that happiness to others.

Your feelings connect you with the knowing and consciousness of your essence. This feeling attribute is essential and must be given to your affirmations. It means you feel, accept, and know it is the truth.

To get results, you cannot be lackadaisical and repeat the claim as if you are reciting the alphabet. Instead, you must speak the words of the affirmation from the solar plexus, where emotional power resides helping you to connect with your feeling self.

To strengthen your declaration, try visualizing yourself experiencing what you are asking for and accepting that it has already manifested in your life.

At this point, try to stay positive and not have doubts and worries which will negate your intentions. The acceptance of your intentions can be helped by embracing a sense of thanks and gratitude in your affirmation. As a result, a receptive state is created, and a feeling of love and humility is felt because the fulfillment of your affirmative has already taken place.

Making an Affirmation
The following tips will help you to make affirmations, or prayers as powerful statements, enabling you to write and say those that will manifest in your life.

Center yourself by relaxing and taking several full breaths into your abdomen.

Establish a sense of the highest love and spiritual consciousness. You should try to make conscious contact with the Creative Source, as you know it, and let it enter your heart and being.

You must give voice to your intention and develop the pattern that you want to create by speaking the words of your affirmation from your solar plexus with feeling and power. Now, you should express thanks to Creative Source once again.

You release and know that your affirmation is answered in the present moment. Now, you can relax, knowing that it is being accomplished for you.

The creation of your affirmations can be an energetic way of connecting to them. Additionally, you may find the following declarations of benefit:

I am grateful for the beautiful gifts in my life.

I am grateful for the abundance of love and joy in my life.

I appreciate all the blessings I have been given.

I am lucky to have such great friends and family.

I am so thankful for all the opportunities given to me.

I am grateful for the kindness of others.

I am thankful for the little things that make life so much better.

I am blessed to have such amazing people in my life.

I am grateful for the beauty of life.

I am thankful for the moments of joy and peace in my life.

I am grateful for the wisdom and guidance from my Higher Self.

All that I do today will be done with love, joy, and peace, and I am thankful.

You will want to make affirmations part of your daily gratitude practice and gather evidence that they are working for you. Share your discovery and use of affirmations with others. When you share them with others they will be encouraged and uplifted and want to use them for themselves. They are great spiritual resources for personal growth.

Chapter 11
EXERCISE ENHANCES FEELING GOOD

Exercise and gratitude are linked most positively. When you exercise, you feel better and have a positive attitude. A change and shift in your mental arenas give a different perspective on your experiences. In addition, the feeling of peace and calm allows you to respond in a less stressful way and keeps you calm.

These have been studied for centuries, beginning with ancient Greek and Roman philosophers. They theorized that physical activity and gratitude could be used to promote mental, emotional, and physical health.

In modern times, this relationship has also been studied extensively. The results of these studies have consistently shown that physical activity can reduce stress and anxiety, improve self-esteem and mood, and increase feelings of pleasure and well-being.

In recent years, scientists have also begun exploring gratitude's effects on physical activity. Studies have found that those who regularly practice gratitude tend to engage in more physical activity than those who do not. This suggests that gratitude motivates people to stay active and maintain their exercise routine.

When observed from a relationship perspective, exercise and gratitude are mutually beneficial. The practice of regular physical activity can help to promote feelings of gratitude, while appreciation can help to motivate you to stay active. Therefore, engaging in both can reap the benefits of improved physical and mental health.

One of the definitions of exercise is "bodily exercise for the sake of developing and maintaining physical fitness." However, exercise has a much more comprehensive range of benefits than just for the physical body. There was a time when people thought of exercise as a way of life because movement is a biological necessity. The body is designed to move, and movement benefits in several areas, including the physical, mental, and emotional areas. Plato stated that when there is a lack of physical activity, the good condition of every human being can be destroyed. Physical activity should be systematic or deliberate to save and preserve human beings.

When you exercise on a regular schedule it affects the immune system, and there is an improvement in mental function. It is also a stress reliever and serves as a positive attitude tool. The adverse effect of stress is reduced during exercise, allowing you to forget the problems and irritations of your day.

In addition, removing daily tension through movement and physical activity can create a calming, clear, and focused mindset.

When you take time to exercise, you are establishing self-care practice because you are focusing on yourself and giving your body what it needs for optimal daily performance. So, exercise also gives you a stress management tool to meet the challenges of your everyday experiences.

Through the movement and activity of exercise, you help create balance and relieve emotions such as irritability, anxiety, and depression that surface.

When selecting an exercise to engage in, try to find one or more that you enjoy. If you have chosen an exercise routine that you do not enjoy, you will probably not follow through on a regular schedule. In developing a plan for your exercise routine try to establish one that is a fit for your needs and one that suits you.

There are many types of exercise to incorporate into your movement routine. Consider rhythmic aerobic or cardiovascular exercise with repetitive motions. The large muscles of the body are engaged in these exercises. If you choose stretching or toning exercises, you will create flexibility and decrease muscle tension.

In establishing an exercise routine, you must set goals to monitor your progress. You might set daily or weekly goals that will work well in keeping you on a goal schedule. The completion of all your goals should be made once you have made a schedule. You can begin with three days a week and increase the days as time permits.

The added benefit of exercise includes a well-balanced body equilibrium. A sense of well-being is achieved when endorphins are released into the bloodstream, and muscle tension is decreased in the body. There is a relaxation response that lessens body tension on both a physical and mental level.

In doing exercise movements, the mind becomes clear, allowing for focus and concentration. There is an increase in self-confidence as you meet your exercise goals and begin to feel better and develop a firm and fit body.

When it comes to exercise, you may think you need a gym membership. However, a gym membership is only sometimes necessary for you to get the benefits of exercise. A beginning step would be to take a walk for 30-45 minutes outdoors, which will also allow you to breathe fresh air and observe the beauty of Nature. The activities of running, jogging, swimming, riding a bicycle, and dancing can all be done free of charge. Physical movement is a necessity for health and well-being.

Action Steps
Find an exercise activity that you enjoy.

Understand what you want to accomplish in your exercise program.

Set a schedule for the hours and days to exercise.

Mix up your exercise routine. (Strength training, jogging, etc.)

Break up your exercise routine into 10-minute intervals if needed.

Walking is a great way to increase your physical activity.

Notice improvements to keep yourself motivated.

Keep an exercise journal to record your progress and feelings.

Get an exercise buddy and set times to meet.

Exercise to music.

These action steps are given as suggestions as you entertain the connection between gratitude and exercise. You will feel better about yourself, and the experiences that you have and view others with more appreciation for their presence in your life.

You should keep an exercise journal for seven days and then reward yourself for the progress you have made in completing your goals. It is now time to give yourself a reward for being successful.

Exercise Quotes

If you want something you have never had, you must be willing to do something you've never done.

Thomas Jefferson

Once you are exercising regularly, the hardest thing is to stop.

Erin Gray

Exercise is the kind of movement that is intentional, purposeful, engaging, and exceptional when it comes to health and mental benefits.

Theresa M. Ross

Chapter 12

MUSIC BRINGS PEACE AND HARMONY

Music is part of our lives and gives us peace and harmony. However, the selection of music for some people depends on their mood. They might want to be uplifted, feel the rhythm of the beat in their body, or listen to music before going to sleep. Music is a potent stimulus with a long history of influencing human emotions.

Because of music, people cry, laugh, and shout or might withdraw within themselves and savor the moment they find themselves experiencing. And so, as we explore the history of music, it reveals that it's a vast and fascinating topic spanning millennia and cultures worldwide. Music has been an integral part of human culture since the beginning of civilization. Various influences, from technological advances to cultural and historical development, have shaped its evolution.

The earliest known evidence of music comes from Paleolithic cave paintings in Europe and Africa. People are depicted playing drums and flutes. By the Middle Ages, music had become an integral part of religious services, with Gregorian chants and other liturgical music developed for Christian worship. In the Renaissance, composers such as Josquin des Pres and Palestrina began to explore the possibilities of polyphonic music and the development of new instruments, such as the lute and harpsichord, which broadened the range of the expression available to musicians.

In the Baroque period, composers such as Bach and Handel developed innovative musical forms, including the concerto and the symphony.

In the classical era, Haydn and Mozart expanded the range of musical expression, further developing the sonata, string quartet, and other forms of chamber music.

By the 19th Century, composers such as Beethoven and Wagner helped push music to its current limits, exploring the possibilities of harmonic and tonal expression. Meanwhile, new genres such as blues, jazz, and country were emerging, and the development of recording technology allowed for the mass distribution of music. In the 20th Century, music continued to evolve, with genres such as rock and roll, hip-hop, and electronic music becoming increasingly popular. Meanwhile, composers such as Schoenberg Stravinsky pushed the boundaries of classical music, exploring the possibilities of tonality and other experimental forms.

Today, music continues to evolve, with new genres and styles being created constantly, from traditional folk music to modern pop music.

The design and creation of music are an ever-changing and ever-growing form reflecting the diversity and creativity of the human experience.

The many changes and ways music developed affected the people listening to it. In addition, new forms of music impacted emotions.

In affecting the emotions, a sense of thankfulness occurs due to a calming of the mind and harmony in the body. Each type of music carried with it a definitive effect. Jazz music brought a peaceful and soulful sound that expressed feelings of gratitude.

Folk music, with its lyrics about life, can often be uplifting depending on the words of a song that is set to music.

Classical music is full of emotions and touches the listener's very essence. The movie, "Pretty Woman," comes to mind when Vivian, played by Julie Roberts, reacts to the symphony playing La Traviata. The music moved her to tears.

Pop and Rock music often have an upbeat and optimistic sound perfect for thinking of and expressing gratefulness.

Then there is world music bringing cultural music sound, and finally, the laid-back and peaceful sound of reggae and country music. All the music categories mentioned help with the expression of gratitude.

World music has a wide variety of sounds from different cultures. It can cause the listener to reminisce about safe travel in a foreign country or thankfulness for having met new friends during a trip.

Reggae music has a laid-back and peaceful sound that is great for expressing positive feelings. And country music has a classic and timeless sound that can be perfect for expressing appreciation.

All the music genres described have their way of influencing the listener. The peaceful and soulfulness of jazz and the uplifting sound of folk music can create a feeling of tranquility. The emotions can often be expressed by listening to classical music or pop music's upbeat, optimistic sound.

You should select music that makes you feel good about yourself and thankful for the beautiful gifts that gratitude brings to you.

The gifts that you receive can only be found when you focus your thinking and look for what enriches your life.

Dr. Randolph Stone, Founder of Polarity Therapy says the following about life. According to him "Life is a song. It has its own rhythm of harmony. It is a symphony of all things which exist in the major and minor keys of Polarity. It blends the discords, by opposites into harmony, which unites the whole into a grand symphony of life. To learn through experience is to blend with the whole, it is the object of our being here."

Music has a profound effect on your thoughts, behavior, and actions. You will probably select music that resonates with how you are feeling or how you want to feel. If you feel like you want to dance, you might choose a song by Beyonce, feeling sentimental, Kenny Latimore singing "For You" might be chosen. Let the music lead you to a place of gratitude. Sometimes there are not enough words to express how you feel, however, use music to speak for you.

Both music and colors have a beneficial effect when they are incorporated into the routines of your life. The two of them can inspire feelings of gratitude and make life pleasant and enjoyable. Try to give each one of them a place in your life and take the gifts of relaxation, peace, joy, hope, resilience and so much more that is given to you.

"When you listen to music the rhythms of life come alive." Theresa M. Ross

Chapter 13

FLOWER ESSENCES FOR EMOTIONAL WELL-BEING

Flower essences, also known as flower remedies or botanical essences, are natural remedies made from the vibrational imprint of flowers. They work by capturing the energy and healing properties of flowers and plants, facilitating emotional and spiritual well-being. While commonly used for treating various emotional imbalances, flower essences can also have a profound effect on gratitude.

Gratitude is the practice of acknowledging and appreciating the positive aspects of life. It is a state of being grateful for what you and it fosters a positive outlook on life. Various studies have shown that practicing gratitude can lead to numerous benefits, such as improved mental health, reduced stress, increased happiness, and enhanced overall well-being. Flower essences can augment and amplify these benefits, providing supportive and transformative experiences.

When it comes to gratitude, flower essences work on an energetic and vibrational level, helping to shift consciousness and perceptions. Each flower has its unique energetic signature that corresponds to specific emotions, qualities, or states of being. By using flower essences, we can tap into the vibrational frequency of specific flowers that resonate with gratitude.

For example, the Bach flower essence called "Gorse" is often used to cultivate gratitude. The essence helps an individual shift from a state of hopelessness and despair to one of renewed faith and optimism. By addressing feelings of desolation and encouraging a positive outlook, Gorse can assist in opening the heart to gratitude.

Similarly, the essences "Wild Rose" and "Sweet Chestnut" can be valuable allies in enhancing gratitude. Wild Rose essence encourages a sense of appreciation of life helping individuals access joy and contentment. While Sweet Chestnut on the other hand aids in overcoming emotional despair and turmoil, leading to a deep sense of gratitude and resilience.

When we consider gratitude, a flower essence that can assist in cultivating and deepening this feeling is the "Sunflower" essence.

An essence that encourages comfort and relaxed alertness is Valerian. It can be used when you are having difficulty relaxing the mind and body

Scientific research regarding the specific effects of flower essences is limited. However, the practice of using them has gained popularity due to the numerous anecdotal reports of positive experiences. Many individuals find that flower essences help them cultivate positive feelings.

Dr. Elizabeth E. Botchis, Ph.D., states that "Plants are visionary teachers and healers whose role is to act as an inner guide, speaking directly to the soul in the language of light."

Flower essences can strongly influence gratitude by working on an energetic level, facilitating shifts in consciousness and perception. Individuals tap into the vibrational frequency of gratitude, encouraging a positive outlook and appreciation for life's blessings.

Explore the use of flower essences by purchasing a book on flower essences and exploring the various essences and how to use them. Now, purchase those that appeal to you in strengthening your gratitude for life and the individuals in your life.

Flower Essence Quotes

"Flower essences allow us to see into the soul of things - into ourselves, our world, and all living beings." Lila Devi

"The beauty of a flower grabs your attention, and its essence speaks to your soul revealing you are more than you think you are." Theresa M. Ross

"The vibrations in flower essences help to release us from our human frailty and remind us of our divine origins."

Theresa M. Ross

Chapter 14

ESSENTIAL OILS AND FEELINGS OF THANKFULNESS

Essential Oils have been part of our lives for a long time. Ancient writings and traditions reveal that aromatics were used in religious rituals, treatment of illness, and both spiritual and physical needs. From records dating back to 4500 BC, there is a description of the use of substances with aromatic properties being used for medical applications as well as religious rituals. The people of ancient times wrote of their use of scented barks, resins, and aromatic vinegars being used in temples, rituals, and medicine. The availability of shrubs, trees, and other plants allowed them to be creative and make use of them in unique ways.

The Egyptians gained mastery in the use of essential oils. In many of their temples, hieroglyphics on walls showed the blending of oils and cited numerous oil recipes. They collected essential oils and placed them in alabaster vessels.

Oils were reintroduced into modern medicine during the 19th and 20th centuries. In recent years, essential oils have gained popularity for their potential therapeutic benefits. From relieving stress to boosting energy levels, these plant extracts are believed to enhance physical and mental well-being. When combined with the practice of gratitude, the synergy between essential oils and a gratitude mindset can amplify the positive effects on overall health and happiness.

An essential oil is the aromatic volatile liquid found within many shrubs, flowers, trees, roots, bushes, and seeds. The liquid is usually extracted through steam distillation. The oils (liquid) are highly concentrated and have greater potency than dried herbs due to the process of distillation which makes them very concentrated.

The uniqueness of essential oils is found in their ability to act on both the mind and body. This makes them different from natural therapeutic substances.

The aromatic compounds in essential oils stimulate various receptors in the olfactory system, which is closely linked to the limbic system, the area in the brain responsible for emotion and memory. As a result, inhaling essential oils can elicit emotional responses and trigger memories that can be supported by the essential oils.

Before using essential oils, check in with yourself to determine what you need now. A choice of oils should not be made before you tune into yourself. You will need to be aware of your feelings and emotions. Are you stressed or is there a need for relaxation? Do you have negative thoughts swimming in your mind and need to bring them to shore? Get a pad of paper and script the way you feel. This will give you a visual representation of where you are in the moment.

The benefit of tuning into yourself comes with being good to yourself and listening to your needs.

When you apply an essential blend that's been diffused with a carrier oil or diffusing a specific scent while practicing gratitude you create a sensory connection between the oil and the feeling of gratefulness. Over time, this association can deepen your experience of gratitude and reinforce the positive neural pathways in the brain.

WAYS TO USE ESSENTIAL OILS

There are several ways to use essential oils. You can use a diffuser, inhale oils on a tissue or cotton ball, or massage diluted oils onto your skin. If you are not familiar with the use of oils and their benefits, be sure to follow the recommended guidelines.

Individuals may occasionally experience rashes or allergic reactions. Always skin test an essential oil before using it.

OILS TO CONSIDER

The following oils are simply recommendations for you to begin to explore the types of oils that you might use.

Lavender – One of the most popular and well-known oils for relaxation. It helps relieve mild anxiety, improve sleep, and calm nerves.

Vetiver – Relaxes and calms the mind.

Frankincense – Aids in calming the mind and easing anxiety. The fragrance's influence is found in increasing spiritual awareness, improving attitude, and uplifting the spirit.

Ylang-Ylang - Brings improvement to your mood. It expands your heart and releases anger, jealousy, and other negative emotions.

Bergamot Oil - This oil is a relaxant and reduces feelings of anxiety and nervous tension. It can also fight symptoms of depression like sadness, disinterest, and feelings of helplessness.

Grapefruit - This one is refreshing and uplifting. It can induce relaxation and reduce depression.

There are a variety of oils to select from and test. If you need in-depth information, an aromatherapist will be able to assist you with oil selection to meet your needs.

CONCLUSION

Many individuals have heard of gratitude and the importance of being grateful. However, few consciously practice gratitude behavior. When you practice gratitude, it makes changes in your thought process and helps with the obtainment of the benefits that it has to offer. In embracing the changes there is a marked improvement in health, better relationships, sleep, and a reduction in stress.

Gratitude is not thought of in terms of bestowing gifts. The question becomes "What gifts." And so, gratitude can become an infrequent occurrence because it is not necessarily thought of as having benefits. Yet it is ever-present, and what it offers is readily available.

This book offers a look at activities that you may be engaged in every day, yet not notice the gifts that you are receiving from the activities. Let us start with a positive mindset. This type of mindset gives relaxation, calmness, thankfulness, a shift in perspective, and more.

When it comes to healthy living, gratitude offers good physical health, psychological health, better sleep, and less stress. Your well-being is part of healthy living, so the gifts offered are a continuation of gratitude's gifts. They include happiness, life satisfaction, value on yourself and others whom you place value on, increased motivation, and productivity.

The awareness and observation of appreciating who you are comes with self-gratitude. The gifts in this area include improved self-esteem, enjoyment of who you are as a person, lower stress, and better days.

There is a connection between self-gratitude and the relationships that you form with others. The appreciation you have for yourself is extended to those with whom you have a relationship. You will experience more satisfaction with your life. There will be greater happiness and relationship commitments.

Your creative talents will be expressed with journaling, causing relaxation, a way to shift to positive and uplifting thoughts. Journaling will help to sharpen your memory and improve your learning ability. There are several types of journals to choose from, so be sure to select one or several that you would enjoy using in your practice. Colors can and should be combined with your journaling, your environment, and your wardrobe. Colors impact your mood, inspire good decision-making, and influence how you think.

Gratitude and mindfulness bring peace and joy into your life. This helps you to recognize and appreciate life's beauty, even when facing challenges. When practicing mindfulness and gratitude together, you can better understand yourself, your relationships, and the world around you.

When it comes to an expression of positive emotions, improved mental health, reduced stress, and increased resilience, think of developing and using affirmations.

The gifts received from gratitude when you exercise are a positive attitude, a feeling of peace and calm, a reduction in stress and anxiety, improved self-esteem, and mood, and an increased feeling of pleasure and well-being.

When you listen to music, your emotions are affected, and a sense of thankfulness is experienced due to the calming of the mind and harmony in the body. The selection of the right kind of music is key.

The addition of flower essences and essential oils to your gratitude toolbox can offer great benefits. These include the power to impact your emotions and feelings of well-being.

There is a connection between all the activities that are given in this book. In many instances, the gifts offered are the same and related to each other. The value of gifts comes in both psychological, physical, and spiritual areas of life. Gratitude offers powerful gifts, waiting for you to take hold of each one that is offered to you. Become aware of ways to be thankful as you experience your daily activities. You will begin to have more peace of mind and gain greater resilience in the face of challenges. With a new perspective, you will have greater emotional strength and a positive mindset.

Look for the gifts of gratitude in every aspect of your daily life. There will be a shift in how you feel, how you relate to others, and the development of a greater appreciation for who you are as a person and your experiences.

BIBLIOGRAPHY

Alvarez, Bella. (2023). *Music Impacts Health in More Ways Than You Think.* https://facty.com/mind/ music-impacts-health-in-more-ways-than-you-think/

Meg Jenkins. (2022). *Mindful Eating a Path to Gratitude and Joy.* https://www.azurestandard.com/azure-life/ blog/mindful-eating-a-path-to-gratitude-and-joy/ c8BeL23v4DrnfcSu

Chelle. *How to Start an Art Journal Step by Step.* (2018). https://artjournalist.com/how-to-start-an-art-journal/

azurestand.com, Mindful Eating a Path to Gratitude

Ballantine, Rudolph, M.D. (1998). *Science of Breath: A Practical Guide.*

Botchris, Elizabeth E. (2017). *Awakening the Holographic Human.*

BrainyQuote.com, 2001-2024.

uhs, Berkeley.edu, University Health Services, Gratitude and Mindful Eating, 2022

Cherry, Kendra. (2020). *What is Meditation?* The what, why, and how. https://chopa.com

Bringing Gratitude to Our Food System. (2017). www. crystalhealingritual.com/crystals

Camille. (2023). *12 Crystals and stones for gratitude.* https://www.crystalhealingritual.com/page/4/?s=12+crystals+and+stones+for+Gratitude

Wright, Kristin Webb. (2023). *Journaling for beginners: how to get started in 10 steps. https://dayoneapp.com/blog/journaling/*

Emmons. R. A., McCullough, M.E.(2003). Counting blessings vs burdens: an experimental investigation of gratitude and subjective well-being in daily life. *Journal of Personality and Social Psychology*, *84*(2), 377–389. https://psycnet.apa.org/doi/10.1037/0022-3514.84.2.377

GoodhouseKeeping.com, 30 Motivational Workout Quotes 2023

Gratitude Grows with a Journal. (2023). https://www.howlifeunfolds.com/search/Gratitude%20Grows%20with%20a%20Journal

Hurley, D. B., Kwon, P. (2012). *The effects of gratitude on music preference and mood.* Psychology of Music.

Johnson Sherrie. What is Self-Gratitude and How Can You Practice It? blog/Self-Gratitude 2022.

Kaplan. The Gratitude Diaries, 2015.

Katz, M & Kaminski P. Flower Essence Repertory: A Comprehensive Guide to North American and English Flower Essences for Emotional & Spiritual Well-Being, 1994.

Latham, Irène & Charles Waters. Dictionary for a Better World, Poems, quotes and Anecdotes from A to Z. Carol Rhoda Books: Minneapolis Hewitt, S., 2020.

Life Science Publishing, Essential Oils Pocket Reference, 2011

Moss L & Moss, M., Wesnes K., Modulations of Cognitive Performance and Mood by Essential Oil Lavender, Pharmacology, Biochemistry and Behavior, 2008

O'Connell, & B. H. O'Shea, D., "An Exploration of the Relationship between music therapy and gratitude "Journal of Music Therapy, 2015

Okeefe, Stephanie, PhD, Improving Relationships Through Gratitude, 2017

Pasricha, Neil, Book of Awesome, 2011

https://www.psychologytoday.com/us/blog/what-mentally-strong-people-don't-do, 2015

Researchgate.com, The Relationship Among Gratitude, Self-Esteem, Social Support and Life Satisfaction Among Undergraduate Students, 2015

Serdar, K'oruk, The Effect of Self-Esteem on Student Achievement, May 2017

Silva, Emily, Sunrise Gratitude, 2020

https://www. Smarterself-help.com, 7 Ways to Express Gratitude in your Relations, 2020

Upperhand.com April 2021

Welch Pamela, M.A., The Energy Body Connection, 2020

INDEX

endorphins 74

essential oils 85

eudaemonic 6

exercise routine 74

F

flower essences 82

folk music 79

formal meditation 64

foundation 63

Fox, Glenn 13

Franklin, Benjamin 41

Freeman, Lyna 62

G

generosity 22

Gibran, Kahlil 46

gifts of appreciations 5

Gilovich, Thomas 25

M

N

U

University of Manchester 13

US Dept. of Health and Human Services 12

W

Wagner 78

Waldinger, Robert 38

Webster Dictionary 1, 41

Winfrey, Oprah 41

Wittenburg, Kaya 33

World Health Organization 11

world music 79

BOOK DESCRIPTION

Discover the transformative power of gratitude with this inspiring new book, *The Gifts of Gratitude: Discover the Power of Giving Thanks.*

Filled with practical advice and wisdom, this book explores the numerous ways in which gratitude can improve our lives. From boosting our mood and reducing stress to increasing resilience and improving relationships. Whether you are facing challenges or simply looking to cultivate more joy and fulfillment in life, the gifts of gratitude are always easily accessible when you want to express them.

You will learn to think about your experiences positively as you think about them.

ABOUT THE AUTHOR

Theresa M. Ross, Ph.D. is an ordained minister, spiritual practitioner, wellness coach, spiritual response practitioner, life coach, and reiki master. She has a special interest in mind, body, and spirit connections. She has always been interested in viewing life experiences from a positive perspective. She applies the lessons learned from great philosophers about beliefs and thoughts that impact one's daily life. This has given her the expertise to help others shift their perspective for a life of joy and peace. She loves to read, write, travel, and spend time outside. She lives in Ann Arbor, Michigan.

MY GIFT TO YOU #1

I have a Gratitude Check Sheet to help you

monitor your Gratitude behavior.

Go to this email address to get a copy.

begrateful89@aol.com

MY GIFT TO YOU #2

It's always rewarding to have a reminder

about gratitude. This small poster has gratitude

quotes on it. Frame it and hang it on a wall as

a daily reminder of the power of gratitude.

Go to this email address to get a copy.??

begrateful89@aol.com

THANK YOU

Thank you for reading my book. I greatly appreciate your interest.
If you want to contact me, please send your message to <u>begrateful89@aol.com</u>.

I would love to hear any comments, questions, or suggestions you may have about this book. I learn so much from my readers and I value our communications.

I am interested in hearing your ideas for new reading material. I strive to make my writing and teaching relevant to you and your journey.

Thank you,

Theresa M. Ross